Why Laughter Yoga or
The Guitar Method

Dedicated to Andrea and Jonas

Walter Birklbauer

Why
Laughter Yoga?

or
The Guitar Method

A Neurological View

Production and publishing:
Books on Demand GmbH, Norderstedt

Email: laugh@laughteryoga.eu

ISBN: 978-3-8423-6907-8

Content

Introduction

As you read the title of this book you might have asked yourself: laughing is ment to be the new magic formula for a better life? Laughter – a remedy for depression? Laughter – a remedy for high blood pressure? Laughter – a remedy for chronic pain? Laughter - an Anti-Aging program? Laughter – a preventive measure for conflicts? Laughter – the answer for Peace on Earth?

Beyond that, don`t we laugh enough as it is? Aren`t we flooded with laughter-provoking offers all day? It starts in the morning radio-shows, where we are confronted with one laughter stimulus after the other.

But this is exactly the point: we have learned to laugh only for a special reason!

Somebody who can be amused quickly is even seen as somebody who has a low intellec-tual capability. And it is even more than that: not only have we learned to interlink laughter with a cognitive trigger, we have learned to act as human beings according to how much social reward and acceptance we receive. So we only laugh for a special reason, as well as we only love for a special reason. We only allow ourselves to be happy if there is a special reason for happiness. But is this really necessary?

This book wants to reach those pragmatic humans, who do not allow themselves to have positive thoughts, a beautiful fantasy or a fulfilling imagination – just for the sake of it.

During my research in the field of individual and social self-controlling I payed much attention to the subject of resource-stimulation on a neuro-somatic level. This also lead me to the most positive and effective form of resource-stimulation – to Laughter Yoga.

This book is meant to help the reader to improve the attitude to "game" and "simulation". It gives an answer to the question why it makes sense to actually spend time in order to activate positive resources. Why should we act "just as if"? And why out of all possibilities "Laughter Yoga"?

I invite the reader to follow my arguments which will lead to a positive attitude towards Laughter Yoga.

What is Laughter Yoga?

Laughter Yoga includes many things, but it definitely excludes one feature: it is not entertainment. Furthermore it is neither religious nor political. It does not fit the atmosphere of a fair or public festival. Laughter Yoga is too serious as to be laughed at.

There is obviously no trademark on "laughing", but there are a few "Laughing-Pioneers", such as Norman Cousins or Patch Adams. And there is the Indian Doctor, Dr. Madan Kataria, who was the first person to pour the act of laughing into a kind of mould and to develop a practical "Users manual". What Bill Gates did for Windows, Dr. Kataria did for Laughter. Based on a series of tests he found out, that the reasons one has for laughing are being overemphasized. On the contrary: he found out, that laughing is possible without a reason, or a joke, or a special sense of humour.

Physical Aspects

The term "Laughter Yoga" (or Hasya-Yoga) is based on traditional Yoga-Breathing-Techniques, as well as special Laughter-Exercises.

By doing this, the neuro-somatic system of a human being stimulates positive emotions. At the same time laughter is one of the best breathing-exercises, because irregular exhaling reduces the oxygen remaining for breathing and so the oxygen-transport is increased even to the level of the cells.

And – without doubt – an optimal cell-metabolistic system is a good basis for a healthy and smooth metabolism of the entire body. So the laughter-exercises have at least two benefits: they intensify the process of exhaling and they stimulate laughter.

At the beginning of the exercise the breathing-aspect is more the centre of focus as opposed to "real" laughter. But as it continues "real laughter" becomes more and more the focus. So laughter-exercises are warming up–exercises, whereby the process of "real laughter" increases continually.

Psychical Aspects

But the laughter-exercises do not only fulfil a physical function by activating feel-good-hormones and reducing stress-hormones.

Very important aspects of these exercises are the overlapping interactions taking place. For example in form of approximate goals. Every laughter-exercise has its own name.

There is, for example, the "Greeting Laughter", the "Handy Laughter", the "Lions Laughter" and many more. But there is also the "Self acceptance Laughter", or the "Forgiveness Laughter". There is also the kind of laughter exercise that helps us to put our problems into perspective.

All exercises follow the same principle – at the moment of the exercise an existing pattern of everyday-experience is being connected with a positive emotion. This increases the possibility that a new positive pattern can develop on a new level of awareness.

Many people for example know the feeling of anger when they see a traffic-jam. At the moment of the awareness of such a situation the limbic system of the brain is automatically activated. This happens so quickly, that it makes no sense trying to think about it or to regulate it, as the emotion of anger is very dominant in this moment[1]. Depending on the individual, this anger will develop a tendency to escalate or de-escalate, or it will develop an awareness for further sources of conflicts.

Laughter Yoga offers a new pattern of reaction in such situations. This new reaction-pattern will be present more and more in experiencing Laughter Yoga. It must however be initiated at a very early point, as the effort of "re-programming" increases continually as soon as one emotion is installed.

The very special aspect hereby is that all these exercises activate our subliminal patterns, which are unconscious. Brain research has shown that our brain continues to learn, even when it is not directly occupied with a current thought or theme. As the brain continues to work in the background as well as during our dreams, it is constantly working on the reorganisation of the neuralgic system.

By doing this it is occupied with all preventive, healing and therapeutic aspects and processes.

---

1 cf. Birklbauer 2007, p. 74, see "Disney-Effekt"

Laughter is not just laughter, it integrates itself as a positive element into the complete physical process of learning. So laughing is not just a pleasurable experience for the moment, it also increases the chance for longer lasting positive changes in life.

Simulation

Alternatively laughter can in the beginning be kindled artificially with a match. Once the glow of the fire is awakened the question of its origin is of no relevance. Human beings work the same way: the body cannot distinguish whether laughter has a "real reason" or not.

When practicing Laughter Yoga the simulation, the "doing as if" works in two kinds of ways: either it works "bottom-up" initiated in the body, or it works "top-down", from the cognitive origin. As neither direction is a "one-way-path" they are a wonderful complement.

"Fake it until you make it….."

….is an essential motto of the Laughter Yoga movement. Here we already touch the key-term for the following explanations. The next chapters describe the benefit of simulation, in the "fake" the "doing as if".

Neuronal patterns of excitement

In scientific studies we find more and more contributions dealing with the positive effect of laughter on mind and body.

"Lachen ist gesund", a German proverb meaning "laughing is healthy" seems to be more than a saying. But is this really the case? Which argument is there that it simply cannot be other than this, or that the chance for the opposite evidence is minimized?

Well, in my explanation I follow the model of the German Psychologist Klaus Grawe. Two of his "life-themes" were the neurologic immunology and neuroscans. One of his primary conclusions refers to the "neuralgic excitement patterns".

He says:

> *"Whenever we feel, think or do something, we do it on the basis of neuralgic patterns of excitement. For everything we experience or do depends*

> *on the fact that specific neurons are*
> *evoked, how fast they are evoked and*
> *in combination with which other neu-*
> *rons they are evoked."[2]*

This hypothesis in no way reduces the complexity of human beings. Mozart`s music cannot be reduced to a plain process of vibrations or binary magnetic conditions. Nevertheless it has an important influence, as every change in the binary set-up has an influence on how we experience music.

Does this mean that Mozart is less fascinating just because I can read the sheet of music? Does the starry sky lose its romantic aspect because scientific knowledge has withdrawn its magic?

Grawe himself draws a good comparison:

> *"Just as the theory of evolution does*
> *not reduce us to apes, so the findings*
> *of neuro-science do not reduce us to a*
> *mere bundle of matter."[3]*

---

2 Grawe 2004a, p. 44

3 Grawe 2004a, p. 58

Cellular activity provides the basis of the emergence which constitutes the very music of our lives. An emergent product can be defined as any quality which could not be explained adequately solely on the basis of its individual constituent parts.

Water is wet, the single water-molecules are not. The feature "wetness" is therefore emergent, as it only arises due to the assembly of many water-molecules.

The quality of our experience can be understood as the emerging result of non-linear interaction of neurones and bunches of neurons, which are registered as physical processes. All patterns of physical processes are reflected in the neuronal patterns of excitement[4]. These are re-activated and repeated since the early days of our childhood and therefore can be triggered easily into a specific emotional direction.

Since we were a child we were learning constantly and we all had experiences which left deep (unconscious) marks on our memory. We

---

4 cf. Grawe 1998, p. 265, quoted after Storch 2002, p. 290

learn if we can reliably count on somebody when we are in need of comfort and security. If a child seldomly experiences a relaxed, balanced atmosphere, well-being or comfort, it will be on a high anxiety-level, which has strong influence on the forming of his character.

All information entering the body through our senses is being transmitted into bioelectric impulses. Our brain is specialized in using these – neurotransmitters are being produced as a reaction to body-sense-experiences and they are the basis of all neuronal structures.

Positive experiences are memorized within a different neuralgic pattern of excitement than negative experiences. Every basic emotional movement (valence) corresponds to a characteristic neuralgic pattern of excitement, which is mixed with the patterns of excitement of the very moment.

Therefore a generally positive emotional basic feeling influences and produces a different neurological pattern of excitement than a generally negative emotional basic feeling.

Grawe comes to the following conclusion:

"If all psychological processes are based on neurologic procedures, then altered psychological processes are based on altered neurological procedures."[5]

Neurological patterns of excitement are reflections of complex, neuro-chemical processes. According to their dimension they will either follow the direction of stress-hormones or feel-good hormones, which produces a completely different experience and field of learning.

This is so, because there is no moment when there is not a reconstruction of the neurological systems in the brain. According to the genetic basis there is a permanent interaction of neuronal tubes being strengthened, neuro-chemical disposition potentials being added, the number and the effect of the responsible receptors being changed.

Furthermore the synaptic evolution is supported, the transformation of neurotransmitters such as serotonins, cortisole, endor-

---

5   cf. Grawe 2004

phins and enkephalins are either increased or decreased, the components of deoxyribonucleic (DNA) are switched on or off.

The intensity and the frequency of the time spent in specific neuronal states of excitement are the basis for a "process of fermentation" within this system. This process can be increased or reduced according to a modality that is not based on logic.

A human being, who, for whatever reason (usually our belief-system plays an important role), experiences mostly situations with negative valences, will initiate different effects on the metabolic processes and the learning-effects of the neuro-somatic apparatus, than a human being who leads a life with mostly positively influenced situations and valences.

If this pattern is repeated often the brain prepares itself for negative conclusions as a result of the current pattern of experience. This again, in turn, initiates further training and repetition.

So a sensitivity for negative emotions can take place, if it is fed with a growing number of impulses that are added throughout a lifetime. Concerning the development of a child Grawe says:

> *"It continuously takes less stimulus to evoke these (impulses). The synapses become more and more able to transport impulses due to the constant facilitation. The regions of the brain that are concerned with negative emotions develop particularly fast."*[6]

For our purposes the whole point is that these neuronal patterns of excitement are not only the product of the input of our every-day life. They are also fed with neuronal patterns of excitement from the past, which influence our conscious and unconscious ideas and memories. Existing neuronal patterns of excitement are either stabilized or reorganized according to their tendency of organisation and order.

Does this mean that patterns of neuronal excitement can be initiated by simulations, for example due to memories, imagination

---

6 Grawe 2004

and inner concepts? Can a positive fantasy be materialized in our body?

The following chapter wants to point out, how these patterns of excitement are directly influenced by our imaginations, memories and inner concepts.

The tube

Due to modern methods of brain-research is has become possible in the last years to make inner processes visible on a cellular level. According to the latest findings a completely new interpretation of our grey matter activities is possible and leads to an upheaval in the field of neuro-science.

Not so long ago, for example, the thesis was relevant, that nerve cells are not able to grow as the brain was seen as a static organism. In the last years, however, the plasticity of this organ was more and more recognized. The field of psychotherapy has a sceptical eye on neurobiology, as it fears that the brain and the mind are being reduced to electro-chemical reactions.

Due to this aspect it is especially interesting that it was a neurobiologist who explained at the 51st Psychotherapy-Congress in Lindau that *"the soul forms the matter of the brain"* [7].

This neurobiologist was Prof. Gerald Hüther from Göttingen and his most important thesis concerned the neurological plasticity of the brain. He described how the experience of an individual with its environmental communication effects the flexibility of neurones and the metabolism of the brain.

Neuronal connections seem to work like a muscle, which diminishes when not demanded, and becomes stronger with intensive training[8]. Through continual transaction with one´s environment a structure is being formed in the "emotional memory" creating successful and unsuccessful coping strategies[9].

Due to modern specialized methods scientists are able to observe the brain as it activates these sectors. Modern technologies such as Magnetic Resonance Imaging (MRI) and

---

7 Rogosch 2001
8 cf. Groenewold 2005
9 cf. Hüther 1996

Positrons-emission-tomography (PET) make it possible to safely depict the function and structure of the brain.

These modern methods are not only able to picture the flexibility and the plasticity of the brain, they can also show the effect of mental processes.

"It is possible to watch the brain at work", were the words of neurobiologist Manfred Spitzer from Ulm, *"while somebody is praying Psalm 23 once with adore, and once without."* It is possible to observe the neuronal patterns which are influenced by our perceptions, physical movement, cognitive achievements and emotions[10].

Spitzer adds:

> *"It is possible to watch the conglomeration of neurons while they are processing new input."*[11]

The prefrontal cortex plays a major role in emotional processes. This has to do with its special neuro-anatomical connection to the limbic system controlling of emotions and

10 cf. Mainzer 2005, p. 8
11 Spitzer 2000, p. 86

behaviour. The left-frontal sector represents positive emotional experiences and the system of approach, whereas the right-frontal sector represents negative emotional experiences and a system of retreat[12].

The outstanding relevance of these constellations is described in a study by Rosenkrantz and others, where a definite connection between the prefrontal cortex and the immune system is found. In this study the test persons where asked to remember the happiest moments and the most terrible moments in their life. Brain-activities was registered before and after this memory. Immediately after this procedure the participants got a vaccination against influenza and the status of the antibodies was checked continuously during the next six month. The result was, that those test persons who had shown strong activity in the left side of the prefrontal cortex while remembering happy moments in their life had produced a lot more antibodies than the other group[13].

---

12 cf. Birbaumer & Schmidt 1999, Davidson 1995, quoted after Debener 2001, p. 9
13 cf. Rosenkrantz et al. 2003

Another investigation, which examined Buddhist monks while meditating with a magnetic resonance scanner also showed an almost constant activity of the left prefrontal cortex. This can be seen as the definite presence of positive feelings[14].

A team of scientists examined 20 test persons with the help of a magnetic resonance scanner. They had all been practicing Buddhist meditation daily for many years.

The result showed that meditation strengthens certain parts of the cerebrum and thereby changes the physical structure of the brain. This was not the case in the brain of people who do not meditate[15].

Studies in the past had already shown a strong activity of the prefrontal cortex in combination with emotional experiences have the following effect: the left frontal sector was activated by experiences creating positive emotions, whereas the right frontal sector was activated by experiences creating negative

---

14 cf. Flanagan 2003, p. 44
15 cf. Gray et al. 2005

emotions. But meanwhile these results are also confirmed by illustrative methods such as PET or fMRI[16]. These methods are of great benefit to science, as they can make visable the brain activity during emotional processes.

With the help of PET it is possible to identify the regional activities of the brain metabolism through so-called PET-scans after injecting a radioactive substance. Energy consumption of the neurons, as well as the change of the regional blood-circulation can then be seen[17].

Due to these developments science can today gain insight into it is today possible to seek information about the dynamics of our internal world with an exactness that has never been possible before.

The American Brain researcher Antonio Damasio was able to localize with the help of PET where in the brain activities occurred, according to whether his test-persons were reminded of happy or sad moments in their

16 Debener 2001, p. 14 ff.
17 cf. Pinel 1997, quoted after Baumann et al. 2005, p. 176

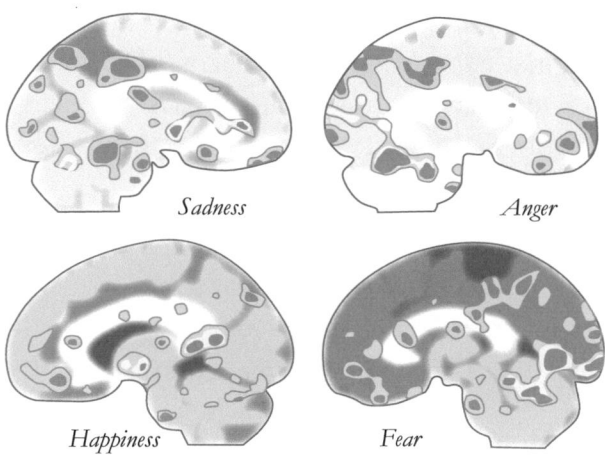

Fig. 1. Happiness and anger in the brain scan

life. To do this he used the positron emission-tomograph (Fig. 1)[18].

According to Damasio the memory of a certain experience, activates not only the sensoric information, but also the physical and emotional data at the time of the experience[19].

When test-persons are scanned during positive or negative memories, the brain tries to reactivate the neural excitement-patterns, as

---

18 cf. Damasio et al. 2000, p. 1050
19 cf. Storch 2002, p. 287

well as the neuro-chemical reactions of the original experience. This means, that an earlier regional state of excitement is stimulated due to the present condition of the context. Damasio says:

> *"The permanent presence of emotions leads to an important consequence: that almost every imagination – no matter if it is experienced at the moment, or it is experienced in memory – is accompanied by some kind of reaction of the emotional apparatus."*[20]

According to Professor Hüther our fantasies and imaginations have a life-long impact on the plasticity of the brain, which is "fed" by our experiences[21].

Scientific progress shows what Physical therapists have been saying all along: that psychological processes are always related to physical consequences. No matter if memories, fantasies or imaginations are conscious,

---

20 Damasio 2006, p. 77
21 cf. Kosslyn et al. 2001, quoted after Milz 2005, cf. Hüther 2004

unconscious, positive, or negative – they are always related to a reaction of the body.

The difference to earlier times is this: in the past we had to believe this is so, now we know it for a fact.

The fertilizer of true sense

If memories and imaginations can indeed produce physical reality, then this revolutionary raw material must be refined[22].

Neuronal excitement patterns can be activated by simply pretending that certain experiences are being made. The stimulation of memories, fantasies or visions is enough to activate stress hormones, as well as opiates or endorphins which are being produced by the body. So it is possible for a positive thought to materialize.

> *The fantasy becomes reality through the reality of the fantasy. (W. B.)*

This means that every positive mental influence redesigns our neuronal network: some-

---

22 Gottwald 2006, p. 16

thing "meaningless" applied in a meaningful way is turned into concrete matter.

So everything that triggers a positive neurological pattern of excitement is to be encouraged and can be used as a resource. This means that it makes sense to reserve time during which our only aim is to produce endorphins, no matter what we do to achieve this.

Here it is not of importance if things are real, the only thing that counts is the reality of the endorphins. Whenever success in the job, a nice bath, a creative experience in the garden, a positive thought, a fantasy, a vision, an inner film, or anything else which is better than expected evokes a positive neuronal pattern of excitement, it can be seen as a positive resource.

A meditation is more than just a meditation, it is a resource. When we imagine something pleasant while meditating, positive neuronal excitement patterns are evoked as if it were real. Pipelines are being built, connections are being looked for, dopamine is produced, electric circuits are edited and the neuro-anatomical structure is being changed.

Even though the simulation is unreal, the body-reaction is real.

Which conclusion can we draw from this? The opiates which are being produced by the body such as endorphins are not dependent on a hundred percent realisation of an urge. Neurological circuits are not dependent on being activated by complex practices, which may come at a high cost to the environment. It is of no importance to them why they are being trained, it is only of relevance that they are being trained at all.

If endorphins can be stimulated by fantasy, there is no longer a need to live the fantasies in real life. The game, the simulation loses the stigma of being artificial. The game is won the moment when we feel something, not only when we have actually experienced it.

When shamans and medicine-men appear in western eyes simply to dance around an ill person, there is a deeper sense to this ritual: to activate the person to stimulate the production of opiates, to strengthen his hope and his will to lead a satisfying life.

When participants of a management training are told to behave in a crazy manner and to try out things they would not usually do, the aim is to let them experience the neuro-chemical state of release from conventional normative rules.

The objective is the simulation of "border-crossings" and the stabilisation of this experience on a neuro-chemical basis. When we speak of release, we speak of neurotransmitters, messenger substances and opiates which are produced naturally in the body and are being released.

It is as if things seem to turn up side down – the "useless" game becomes an important instrument by scanning the "hot spots" of the body which are in the background or decoded in a special way. Nonsense turns into the source of coming to one`s senses. Chaos becomes the detective of our unconscious.

So it happens that the act of laughing is all of a sudden not only funny, it also makes sense surprisingly enough. So all of a sudden there is sense in laughing without a reason. Because then laughter is like embalming our soul and is new energy for the present.

Nonsense becomes the fertilizer of sense! "Senselessness" evokes the production of endorphins which have their source in the very individual history of every person. This stimulates the "exploitation of natural resources" which are hidden in the depth of our soul.

Laughter is the simplest method of giving a positive input to the way we experience our life. It can also be seen as the best initiator for a continued process of fermentation.

Artificial laughter is like tickling a smile. The playful "doing as if" laughter can be compared with a small safety parachute which is there only to make sure that the main parachute opens at the right time.

The Guitar Method

The title of this book is "Why Laughter Yoga?". The title could just as well be "Why positive thinking?", "Why meditation?", "Why primal-scream-therapies?". There has been strong demand for happiness and wellbeing in the last years. A strong economic boom is the result, one can also call it the "doing as if" boom. Books about happiness present happiness-recipes, artificial beaches are created in huge swimming-arenas, seminars in neurolinguistic-programming teach how to set emotionally effective anchors.

Time-Management, relaxation-techniques, Zen-archery, meditation, mental training, autogenic training, "explore yourself" courses, yoga, seminars about a satisfying life and the ideal diet – all these offers have the same aim and focus on different sources.

It does not seem to be of great importance which method is being used, they are all successful as long as they manage to evoke *positive neuronal states of excitement.*

Now we could develop these thoughts further on. If all these methods are effective, we could also invent our own method and test it. My suggestion is to simply invent "The Guitar Method" spontaneously. An important point of our "Guitar Method" is, that each assumption, each simulation, each imagination, each memory moves something within us - this is

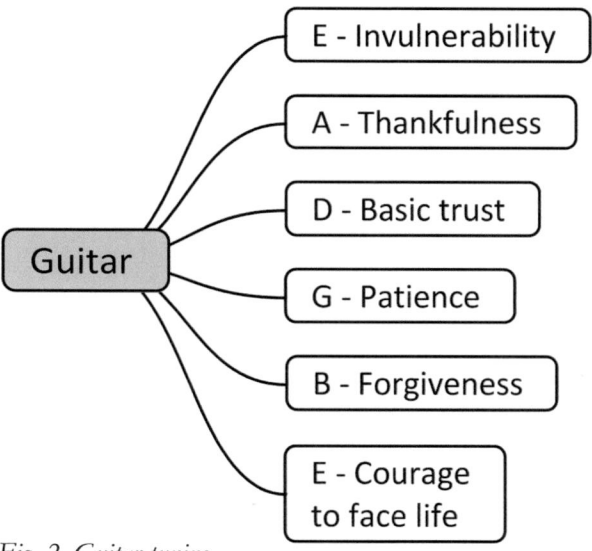

Fig. 2. Guitar tuning

based on the contents of the previous chapters.

Tune versus perfection

First we could decide to take some time in the morning to pitch ourselves - like we would pitch a guitar before playing it. The thought behind is that any chord, played on guitar that is not in tune, cannot be effective, even if it is played perfectly. On the other hand, if we have a true guitar, we can play a chord on it even technically not perfectly and it will still sound okay. For our daily routine this means that even if have missed the bus in the morning, even if there is no coffee in the office or the traffic lights were red all the time, the sound of the chord is still pleasant if we have pitched the psychological guitar. How can we do that?

Overtones and undertones

The next step is to assign an emotion to each string (Fig. 2 and 3). We could assign the deep E-string to the field of invulnerability, pride and boundaries. Here we can put on the life's accoutrements of knighthood which protect us from the risks of life, the adversarial arrows that come across. It is possible to train strength in life despite the feeling of having a sword of Damocles, which many people have when it goes to invisible dangers like cellular communications or radioactivity.

In daily life we will remain who we are, but now we try to realize the feeling of invulnerability. The better we pitch this string, the better the quality of the chord will be.

We could continue like this now.

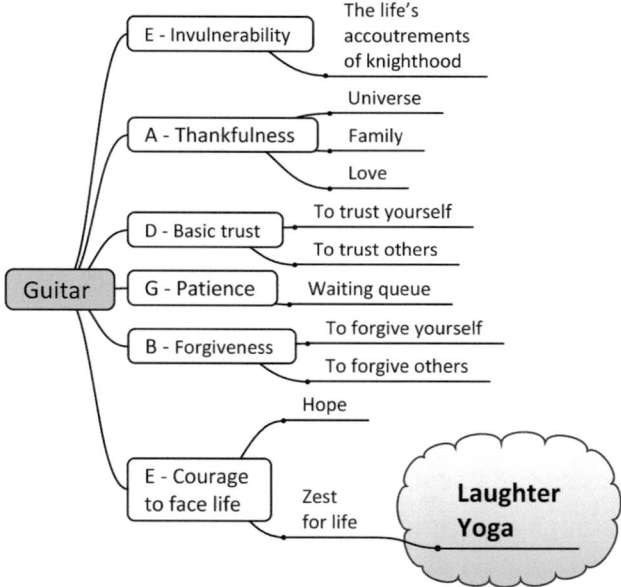

Fig. 3. Laughter Yoga supports zest for life

The A-string could be assigned to the feeling of thankfulness and love - towards the universe and the family. We could fall in love with life like if it was something unreachable.

The D-string could deal with the complex of trust - trust in other persons and in ourselves. The G-string could deal with patience, imagining oneself in a very long cue - as content as possible. To support this imagination, we could add real memories of situations with which we where able to cope successfully. We need not find the perfect memory immediately, we can take any memory and use it as place holder. As soon as we find a better memory, we will substitute it with this one.

The B-string could be assigned to the field of forgiving - forgiving oneself and others. And the E-string could address the courage to face life, with the overtones of hope and joy. The concept of joy offers the possibility to integrate Laughter Yoga.

If you practice the daily pitching regularly, the sound of the chord which arises, can become like a rock or a "house of calmness".

Why Laughter Yoga?

But Laughter Yoga finally is a variable that can be substituted with other methods. And still Laughter Yoga is especially effective, because it activates and conserves positive emotions like no other method and it is bound up with converging aims.

Laughter Yoga changes the present - and the future. It is a massage for the inner organs, it loosens the muscles, strengthens the immune system and decreases chronic pain.

Whereas children laugh approximately 400 times a day, grown ups only manage a mere 15 times. Every "true" laughter eliminates stress for this very moment.

In his research on mimic the American anthropologist and psychologist Paul Eckmann found different varieties of the human smile. 18 ways of smiling are not authentic according to him, they have a strategic aim in human communication.

Only the laughter whereby the "orbicularis oculi" – a muscle around the eyes, is contracted, leads to the so-called "Duchenne Laughter". Many generations of actors have had a hard time with this muscle, as it cannot be contracted by will by a very large part of mankind.

But it can be provoked, without reason. There are two ways to experience true laughter – either you have a good reason for laughing, or you start with a "act as if". Since medical computer are able to give us a picture of different parts of the human being, there is almost nothing which has not been seen in the "tube".

Results of these latest findings are of big help to all scientific fields, also the field of gelotology - the research of laughter. The hypothesis described above, that our brain shows neurological reactions even if it only imagines situations and acts "as if", could be confirmed with x-ray pictures.

Completely different neurological activity patterns in the brain are activated if we have positive thoughts, as opposed to negative imaginations. This means that every positive thought and every positive vision which stimulates the production of endorphins becomes concrete matter.

So this "acting as if" can also be applied to our body experience: we can stimulate "true laughter" by willingly starting with "fake laughter". The "fake laughter" can be seen as starting-energy for the "true laughter".

Laughter Yoga combines the functions of body and mind on a level of "acting as if", and thereby influences us in a psychological, as well as a physical manner. Laughter exercises to provoke relaxation of the body, which has a positive influence on the breathing and the muscles.

On the other hand the laughter exercises activate our psychological "hot spots", because well known reaction patterns are being replaced by a positive body-feeling which is produced with the help of already existing resources.

Laughter can be seen as the most positive way of activating resources of the body, not only in the situation of laughter itself, but also with long lasting effects.

Laughter always produces endorphins, self-produced morphines which inevitably lead to a physical wellbeing. The latest brain-research results point out that it makes sense to reactivate positive resources regularly, as this has a positive impact on the complete neuro-somatic system.

Laughter Yoga is more than simply "laughing". Laughter Yoga aims to re-activate the ability to laugh without losing oneself in the picture of a an ideal world.

How does Laughter Yoga work?

Laughter Yoga helps to increase the times in which one is in a positive emotional state of mind. By doing this, it helps to repeat and reactivate the neuro-somatic positive effects and promotes their long term influence on body and mind.

Laughter Yoga promotes new somatic markers

One of the most elementary components in the work of Damasio`s is the subject of the somatic markers.

Somatic markers are a system of biological evaluation system originating in the prefrontal cortex. Here all signals from the five senses, as well as all other parts of the body are accumulated, they activate fantasy images which then produce feelings[23].

This works due to neuro-chemical states of the body, which have been memorized and can be re-activated through memory or visualisation in form of a fuzzy, blunt recall.

---

23 Somatic markers are measured on the basis of skin resistance; can be found in Damasio 2006, Playingcard Experiment, cf. http://arbeitsblaetter.stangl-taller.at/GEHIRN/GehirnEmotion.shtml

We are talking about body-memories, which are activated by the stimulation of certain feelings, themes, objects or thoughts. Damasio explains, that memorized feelings linked to certain experiences influence our thoughts and our awareness.

> *"If an unwanted result comes to your awareness in connection with one possibility of reacting in a certain situation, then you will have an unpleasant body-feeling, at least for a short time.* [24]

Somatic marker do not record our conscious processes, but also the unconscious mental and physical perceptions, as well as memories, plans and inner statistics which we develop for our assessment of the world.

This means that every experience which evokes associations from the past reanimates us in a neuro-somatic manner, and also conservatively connects us to the future. Due to this an experience- and belief-system about

---

24 Damasio 2006, p. 237

what is "good" and "correct" is being installed on a biological basis.

Laughter Yoga offers a new possibilities to our reaction-systems by connecting laughter with a new inner pattern this is being trained like a muscle. So Laughter Yoga supports new somatic markers.

Laughter Yoga formulates approximate goals

The Zurich Resource concept of Maja Storch and Peter Krause suggests resource-orientated self management. They encourage with objectives which focus on approach, not on avoidance. This starts, for example, with the use of language.

There is a difference if I say: *"I do not let myself be rushed"*, or if I say *"I allow myself tranquility"*. The first option includes the neurological equivalent of a negative potential. Neuro-physically an unwanted state of being is activated. The second sentence allows a vision of a state of being desired. Neuro-physically a positive pattern of excitation is being evoked and this makes the desired behaviour more likely[25].

When positive thoughts are linked with positive emotions, new positive states of excitation are formed and create new patterns of order. If the new order patterns and the equivalent physical processes are repeated continuously new patterns of thinking, feeling and acting are the result. These need to be supported consciously when the process begins.

Laughter Yoga promotes patterns of feeling aroused

As mentioned above, physical processes have an impact on special positive or negative patterns of excitement. Klaus Grave defines "resources" as all activities which combine positive emotions and manners of thinking to a neurological pattern of excitation which is also positive[26].

The best method of altering a neurological pattern of feeling is by slowly replacing the old pattern with a new one. To do this successfully it is not enough to just talk about the

---

25 cf. Storch 2005, p. 12
26 cf. Grawe 1998, p. 445, quoted after Storch 2002, p. 290

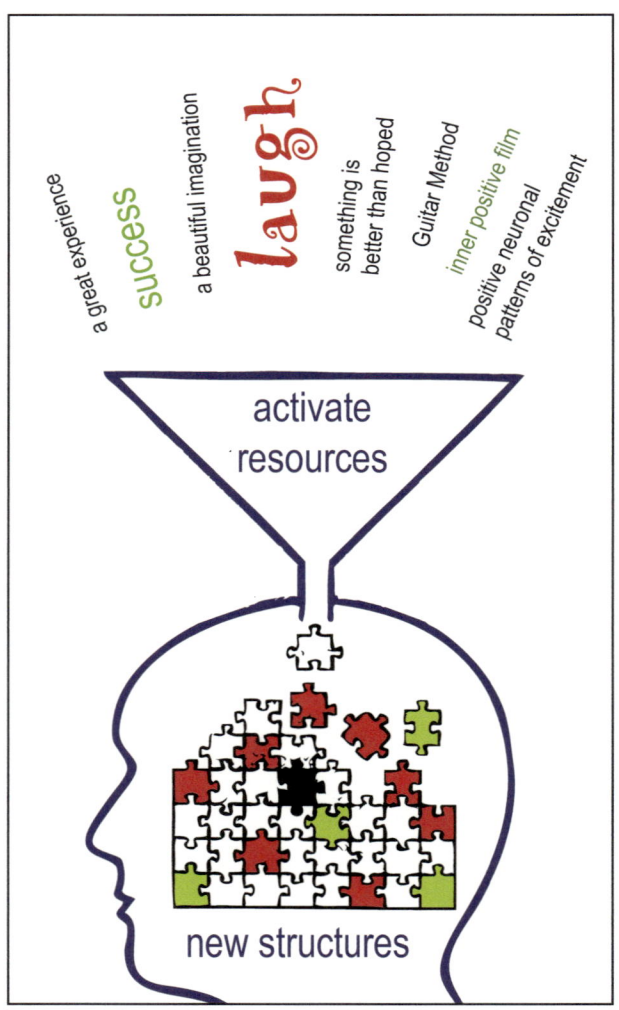

Fig. 4

desired change. There must be interaction in emotional activation, in order to reach a new level of organisation. Laughter Yoga is only one instrument among many, but it is a very effective one, because it provides exactly this interaction. With the help of memory, imagination, fantasy and association in connection with very easy activities such as "Laughter", positive patterns of excitation are practiced.

Laughter Yoga activates resources

The activation of resources leads to a new habits of feeling. In order to change a present pattern of excitation a new neurological net must be activated for so often, that a new pattern automatically replaces the old one[27]. Instruments used to activate resources can be positive thinking, as well as imagination or any kind of positive experience. One of the best "tools" however, to activate specific body-resources is laughter itself (Fig. 4).

Laughing out of full heart and negative stress are mutually exclusive emotional states

---

27 Storch 2002, p. 290

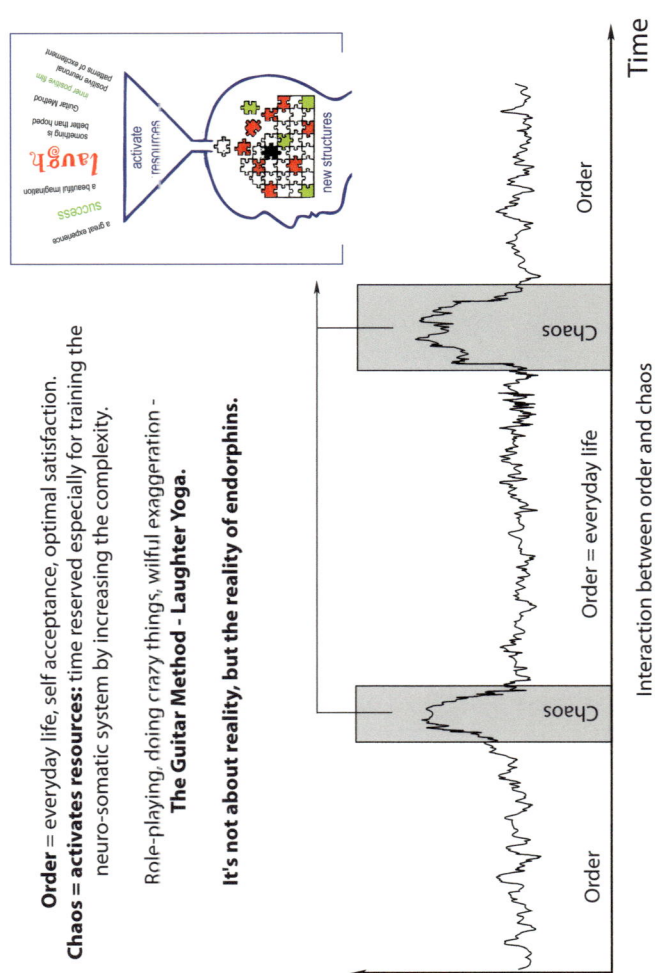

Order = everyday life, self acceptance, optimal satisfaction.
Chaos = **activates resources:** time reserved especially for training the neuro-somatic system by increasing the complexity.

Role-playing, doing crazy things, wilful exaggeration - **The Guitar Method - Laughter Yoga.**

It's not about reality, but the reality of endorphins.

Fig. 5

of being. A person who laughs heartily will always arrive in the present.

A Laughter Yoga session does not only relieve pain at the moment, it has a long-term effect on a person`s mental state and mood in which a person is. Communication, and the ability of approaching people and the relationship to other people in general profit from Laughter Yoga.

Certainly it is not the aim to become a "happiness freak" and only see the world in a pink shadow…

It is not without reason that in the course of evolution cautious humans who were the ones who survived. This, whoever, led to the fact, that those happy humans, who ended up between the teeth of a dangerous fish have died out.

The cautious humans, the ones who are always careful, have survived – but they are the ones who have a default in their brain, which is more adapted to signals of stress than to those of happiness and well-being[28].

---

28 cf. LeDoux 2001, p 22

One more reason to spend time on balancing these parts of the brain. Laughter Yoga is a perfect possibility to do this, a way of spending time where positive resources are being activated and repeated.

This is the time for playing games, for exaggeration, fantasy and emotional supercharge. It is the place where we can learn to be our own friend. It means to practice hard in order to make the best out of it in everyday life. Here we can train our inner autopilot and improve the scarf-skin of life. It is the situation in which nonsense makes sense and chaos is justified (Fig. 5).

Everyday life is a time of survival, giving one`s best, in order to come to a present state where one accepts the current level of satisfaction. This relieves us of the logic of failure in day-to-day life. It also encourages the idea that one is allowed to be just the person one is, and still keep a certain goal in mind.

The impact of Laughter Yoga

The more science explores aspects of laughter, the more evidence is being found. Gelotology – laughter research – even goes so far as to say that laughing increases the number of T-lymphocytes and so-called "helping-cells" and hereby strengthens the immune-system and helps to prevent heart disease.

It makes sense to increase the time spent in a positive emotional states thus improving the basis of non-linear neuro-somatic "fermentation processing".

Research scientists working for Michael Miller at the University of Maryland showed test persons funny films and scenes from the film "Saving private Ryan", measuring the contraction and dilation of the blood vessels of the spectators.

Laughter proved to have an impact on the relaxation of the vessels and on blood circulation. When watching war-movies, however, the vessels of the test persons contracted and blood-circulation was reduced.

So one can imagine what will happen if we repeat such neuro-somatical patterns during our everyday life – it makes no difference if we do this by randomly selected confrontation, by using fantasy, memories, consciously, or unconsciously.

In every case it will have a self-organisation effect in the field of training, learning and repetition.

Aspects of Health

The effect of Laughter Yoga can be categorized in individual and social aspects. The short-term effects of Laughter Yoga on an individual basis are: reduction of stress hormones, change of the emotional status within a short period of time, production of "happiness hormones" and reduction of pain due to endorphins as well as massage of inner organs.

On a long term basis Laughter Yoga reduces states of depression states, it enriches the quality of one`s basic mood, and has positive impact on pulse-frequence, as well as the blood-pressure and the immune system.

Social Aspects

Laughter Yogis become more communicative, which leads to an increase in social interaction. Furthermore laughter Yoga helps to establish a common emotional basis exchange, which leads to an improvement of human relationships, motivation, sense of humour, creativity and communication.

Individual competence is being strengthened which is felt especially in relation to conflict. Personal competence makes better use of one`s resources. This is the basis for a new positive form of interaction within a cultural setting.

On the one hand Laughter Yoga enables forgiveness and letting go. Practicing patterns of forgiveness and linking them with positive emotions, increase that these abilities can be lived more frequently in every-day life.

> *Forgiving means letting go. Letting go means freedom. Forgiving means not to burden the present. From an egoistical point of view forgiving is economical. From an altruistic point of view forgiving is human. (W. B.)*

In a neurological sense this means not repeating the neurological content which is evoked by not forgiving. It is not possible to change what has been, but we can change the approach to the past. This is also a form of forgiving and letting go.

On the other hand, due to a steady repetition of new emotional patterns these can be turned around in a positive direction. In this sense Laughter Yoga can be compared to a life jacket, as is helps to keep conflicts on the surface, rather than letting them be drawn into the depths of other conflict themes. It does not necessarily change the content of the actual conflict, but it influences the way we continue to act in relation to it.

Further positive impacts of Laughter Yoga are: a greater tolerance-level to faults and mistakes – also relating to oneself -, a positive approach to playing as well simulating. The conflict-researcher Friedrich Glasl says that "golden moments" are created by sharing positive memories.

Due to the positive climate in the group cohesiveness is at its optimum. By being integrated in the group one feels part of the community. Due to this group members can develop their maximum talent.

This in turn makes optimal productivity and a spirit of innovation among the group members more likely, possibly leading to the readiness for a modern togetherness.

Field of application

In India the field of application is increasing all the time. Indian policeman are trained in Laughter Yoga, there are successful experiments with Laughter Yoga in prisons, and in schools for the blind students learn Laughter Yoga by using their hands.

But also in the rest of the world there are more and more reports about Laughter Yoga. In the strongly disciplined Japanese Society Laughter Yoga almost has a soul-freeing effect. In homes for elderly people Laughter Yoga is used to conjure a smile on the faces of the people in a magic kind of way.

In Firms and organisations Laughter Yoga is practiced regularly to reduce stress and positively effect the working-climate.

Theatre Groups use Laughter Yoga as warm-up exercise to reduce tension. Seminars lasting one or more days practice Laughter Yoga to build up a strong emotional basis, as well as a positive atmosphere more quickly.

I can think of the following areas where Laughter Yoga could also be integrated: in families, preventively in intercultural fields, before tests or exams in teaching environments, in medical fields, where the daily experience on the job is in contrast to that of private life.

Laughter Yoga Sessions

The main aim of this book is not to give detailed instruction for Laughter Yoga. The focus lies on the "why Laughter Yoga", rather than "how Laughter Yoga". This is why it only illustrates a Laughter Yoga Session in a very condensed way.

According to Dr. Madan Kataria a Laughter Yoga Session is divided into three parts. It begins with an introduction, followed by laughter-meditation, ending with a relaxation-phase for mind and body, also referred to as Yoga-Nidra-Session.

Introduction

When going to theatre or to the opera, we usually clap our hands in an ordinary sort of way. This is different when practicing Laughter Yoga.

Here our hands are brought together with fingers slightly apart. This stimulates the acupressure points in the palm of the hand. While clapping we follow this beat:

1 2 – 1 2 3

Then we replace numbers with letters and the following words:

Ho Ho – Ha Ha Ha

Then a breathing exercise is introduced: we bend our body forward, taking a deep breath while coming into an upright position again and then stretching the arms above our head. Laughter accompanies the breathing out.

The last exercise of the introduction is meant to waken the child within us by clapping our hands twice, calling: "very good, very good – yeah" and stretching our arms up into the air.

Laughter Yoga Exercises

The session usually starts with "Welcome Laughter". We fold our hands like in the Indian "Namaste", look into each others eyes and laugh. Then we proceed to the next person.

"Chilli Laughter" is the kind of laughter where we imagine having eaten something very hot and try to get relief by fanning fresh air to the mouth with our hand. Eye contact is very important. Eye contact and laughter are the keys to real laughter.

"Lion Laughter" relaxes our face-, eye- and neck- muscles. We open our eyes, stick out the tongue, hold our hands next to the ears with the palms facing outward – similar to the palms of a lion coming towards you - and we laugh. It is important to laugh, not to roar.

One of my favourites among paradox interventions is the "Argument Laughter". Hereby we raise the right or left hand and gesticulate with our index finger as if we were angry at somebody. This is finger wagging not with to a feeling of anger, but with laughter. It can provoke true miracles when driving the car!

One more favourite is "One Inch Laughter". We show the person standing in front of us that the reasons for being angry are very small and of no importance by holding thumb and index finger very close to each other, with a gap of approximately 10 millimetres. Automatically laughter will be initiated, especially when men and women meet.

"Milkshake Laughter" can be practiced standing in a circle without changing partners. Hereby we act as if we would be pouring liquid from one glas into another. After doing this three times the liquid is being poured behind our shoulders accompanied with delightful laughter.

"Triumph Laughter" gives our thymus-gland a good massage and helps us to go through life with a secure grounded feeling. We pound our chest with our fists like Tarzan laughed from the bottom of our heart while doing so.

Self-acceptance is a dominant theme in our days, the ability to laugh about oneself and to be one`s own friend. This can be achieved with the "Laughing about myself Laughter". We point our fingers at ourselves and start to accept and like ourselves, we laugh about our own faults. This is a very important Laughter Yoga Exercise, as it continues its effect in the back of the brain after the session.

Another important topic of our time is "Forgiveness Laughter". We practice – without having a special reason to do so – the pattern of forgiveness. Hereby we open our hands as if we wanted to hold somebody in our arms, we approach a partner, look into each others eyes and laugh. This exercise also has a long-term effect on our brain.

Then the time has come for the so called "Gradiant Laughter", the rising laughter. Similar to the "Milkshake Laughter" this exercise does not need a partner. We stand in a circle or just by oneself and start to laugh very silently and slowly and then gradually get louder – from zero to one hundred. This exercise often gets even the most hesitant participants going.

The Laughter Yoga session can end, for example, with the "Rowing Laughter". Hereby we all sit on the floor, one behind the other. We move our arms as if we were rowing a boat, all following the same rhythm, and counting to three. When leaning back the fourth time we lay our head on the person sitting behind us, while moving the arms up into the air. Due to our head lying on the tummy of the person behind us, the persons laughter-movements also stimulate our own laughter.

Due to the many laughter exercises which have been practiced up to this point, only a small impulse is needed to cause true, durable laughter. Often the waves of laughter can be experienced as arousing each other, with a synergetic effect, becoming stronger, then decreasing again and finally coming to an end.

This is exactly the right time for Yoga-Nidra, relaxation. It is a meditation led by the Laughter Yoga-Coach, whereby a deep relaxation is stimulated by leading awareness to different parts of the body.

Bibliography

Baumann, K., Kessler, H. & Linden, M. (2005): Die Messung von Emotionen. Verhaltenstherapie und Verhaltensmedizin, 26(2), p. 190 - 202.

Birbaumer, N. & Schmidt, R. F. (1999): Biologische Psychologie, edition 4, Berlin: Springer.

Birklbauer, W. (2010): Zeitfusion, Die Selbstorganisation neuronaler Erregungsmuster, BoD.

Damasio, A. R., Grabowski, T. J., Bechara, A., Damasio, H., Ponto, L. B., Parvizi, J., Hichwa, R. D. (2000): Subcortical and cortical brain activity during the feeling of self-generated emotions. Nature Neuroscience 3. 1049 - 1056.

Damasio, A. (2006): Ich fühle, also bin ich. Die Entschlüsselung des Bewusstseins. List: München.

Davidson, R. J. (1995): Cerebral asymmetry, emotion, and affective style. In R. J. Davidson & K. Hugdahl (Hrsg.), Brain asymmetry p. 361 - 387. Cambridge: MIT Press.

Debener, S., (2001): Individuelle Unterschiede in der frontalen EEG-Alphaasymmetrie: Emotionalität und intraindividuelle Veränderungen, Berlin: Dissertation.de.

Flanagan, O. (2003): „The Color of Happiness", New Scientist, vol. 178, 24.05. p. 44 ff.

Gottwald, C. (2006 in print): Körperpsychotherapeutische Perspektiven zur Neurobiologie. In: Marlock G., Weiss H. (Ed.): Handbuch der Körperpsychotherapie. Stuttgart: Schattauer. Internetversion: http://www.eidos.at/inhalt/artikel/neurobio.htm.

Grawe, K. (2004): Von der Verhaltenstherapie zur Neuropsychotherapie? Opening lecture on the 15th Congress of Clinical Psychology, Psychotherapy and Advice from 5. – 9.3.2002 in Berlin. Internet Stand 02/2004: http://www.bvvp.de/news04/vt_nt_grawe.htm.

Grawe, K. (2004a): Neuropsychotherapie, Hogrefe.

Grawe, K. (1998): Psychologische Psychotherapie. Hogrefe: Göttingen.

Gray, J. R., Lazar, S. W., Kerr, C. E., Wasserman, R. H., Greve, D. N., Treadway, M. T., McGarvey, M., Quinn, B. T., Dusek, J. A., Benson, H., Rauch, S. L., Moore, C. I., & Fischl, B. (2005): Meditation experience is associated with increased cortical thickness. Neuroreport. 16(17): p. 1893 - 1897, November 28.

Groenewold, U. (2005): Per Tomographie und Spektroskopie sehen Ärzte, wie eine Therapie das Gehirn psychisch Kranker verändert. Ärzte Zeitung. 16.12.

Hüther, G. (1996): The central adaptation syndrome: Psychosocial stress as a trigger for adaptive modifications of brain structure and brain function. Progress in Neurobiology, 48, p. 569 - 612.

Hüther, G. (2004): Die Macht der inneren Bilder. Wie Visionen das Gehirn, den Menschen und die Welt verändern. Göttingen. Vandenhoeck und Ruprecht.

Kosslyn, S.M., Ganis, G. Thompson, W. L. (2001): Neural foundations of mental imagery. Nature Review Neuroscience. 2, p. 635 - 642.

LeDoux, J. (2001): Das Netz der Gefühle. Wie Emotionen entstehen, München: Deutscher Taschenbuch Verlag.

Mainzer, K.(2005): Was sind komplexe Systeme? Komplexitätsforschung als integrative Wissenschaft. (unpublished manuscript). Augsburg.

Milz, H. (2005): Körpertherapie - an Leib und Seele genesen. Lecture: 1. Grazer Psychiatric - Psychosomatic Conference.

22.1.2005. Internet: http://www.helmutmilz.de/documents/KongressGraz1_05.pdf.

Pinel, J. P. J. (1997): Biopsychologie. Heidelberg: Spektrum - academic publishing.

Rogosch, J. (2001): Wie die Psyche das Gehirn baut. Badische Zeitung, 02.05.2001.

Rosenkrantz, M.A., Jackson, D.C., Dalton, K.M., Dolski, I., Ryff, C.D., Singer, B.H., Muller, D., Kalin, N.H., Davidson, R.J. (2003): Affective style and in vivo immune response: Neurobehavioral mechanisms. PNAS 100: p. 11148 - 11152.

Spitzer, M. (2000): Geist im Netz. Heidelberg.

Storch, M. (2002): Die Bedeutung neurowissenschaftlicher Forschung für die psychotherapeutische Praxis. Psychotherapie, vol. 7, issue 2. p. 281 - 294 CIP-Medien, München.

Storch, M.; Krause, F. (2005): Selbstmanagement - ressourcenorientiert. Grundlagen und Trainingsmanual für die Arbeit mit dem Zürcher Ressourcen Modell (ZRM). 3. revised edition.